Managing Diabetes
A Wholefood Approach

Written by Pauline Byers

No part of this publication may be reproduced, stored in a retrieval system or transmitted in any form or by any means, electronic, mechanical, photographic or otherwise, without the prior permission of the author.
© 2003 Pauline Byers MA BSc RN RM RHV Cert Ed

British Library Cataloguing in Publication Data
A Catalogue record of this book is available from the British Library
ISBN 09531405-9-8

Published by Managing Diabetes
PO Box 5598 Derby DE1 9EQ, United Kingdom
Email: info@managingdiabetes.co.uk
website: www.managingdiabetes.co.uk

Cover design: Beulah Vision, www.beulahvision.net

Contents

What is Diabetes?	1
A Success Story	8
Users' Comments	17
Diet and Lifestyle	19
How to Maximise Blood Sugar The Byers Model	32
Daily Walking Diaries	34
Recipes	
Main Courses	38
Cooking with Tofu	45
Cooking with Rice	53
Cooking with Beans	56
Cooking with a range of Vegetables	62
Breakfast Foods	74
Desserts	80
Tasty Spreads and Dips	91
References	98

Acknowledgments

Thanks to all my friends for their encouragement over the months and for their patience in trying foods cooked in new ways.

Thank you Mollie, your dedication to people is beyond that of most.

What is diabetes?

Diabetes mellitus is a condition in which the amount of glucose (sugar) in the blood is too high because the body cannot use it properly. Insulin is vital for life. It is a hormone produced by the pancreas that helps the glucose to enter the cells where it is used as fuel by the body. The main symptoms of untreated diabetes are increased thirst, going to the loo all the time - especially at night, extreme tiredness, weight loss, genital itching or regular episodes of thrush, blurred vision and excessive sweating.

Types of Diabetes

There are two main types of diabetes. These are:
Type 1 diabetes, also known as insulin dependent diabetes
Type 2 diabetes, also known as non insulin dependent diabetes

Type 1 diabetes develops if the body is unable to produce any insulin. This type of diabetes usually appears before the age of 40. It is treated by insulin injections and diet and regular exercise is recommended.

Type 2 diabetes develops when the body can still make some insulin. This type of diabetes usually appears in people over the age of 40, though it often appears before the age of 40 in South Asian and African-Caribbean people. It is treated by diet and exercise alone or by diet, exercise and tablets or by diet, exercise and insulin injections. The main aim of treatment of both types of diabetes is to achieve blood glucose and blood pressure levels as near to normal as possible. This, together with a healthy lifestyle, will help to improve wellbeing and protect against long-term damage to the eyes, kidneys, nerves, heart and major arteries.
Adapted from**www.diabetes.org.uk/diabetes/under.htm.**

What is the Hb A1C?

The Hb A1C is formed in the blood chemical, haemoglobin. Basically sugar sticks to the haemoglobin to make a 'glycosylated haemoglobin', called haemoglobin A1C or Hb A1C. The more sugar in the blood, the more haemoglobin A1C or Hb A1C will be present in the blood.

Red cells live for 8 -12 weeks before they are replaced. By measuring the Hb A1C it can tell you how high your blood sugar has been on average over the last 8-12 weeks. A normal non-diabetic Hb A1C is 3.5-5.5% (this varies between hospitals). In diabetes 4-6% is acceptable. The Hb A1C test is currently one of the best ways to check diabetes is under control; it is the blood test that gets sent to the laboratory, and it is done on the spot in some hospital clinics.

Remember that the Hb A1C is not the same as the sugar level. Coincidentally the sugar/Hb A1C numbers for good control are rather similar though: sugar levels 5.5-6.5 mls/l half an hour before meals versus 7% Hb A1C. Adapted from **http://medweb.bham.ac.uk/easdec/prevention/what_is _the_hba1c.htm#hba.**

Learning to Manage Type 2 Diabetes

To do this we need to take a careful look at what we eat and this is what this book is all about. **Type 2 diabetes** is a lifestyle disease. That means it is caused by the way we live. Inactivity and too much to eat are the major factors in bringing on this disease. Although some people have inherited a genetic predisposition to develop diabetes, genetics is like a loaded gun, it doesn't hurt anyone unless you pull the trigger. It is a sedentary lifestyle together with a high fat diet that pulls this trigger, bringing on diabetes. By understanding how lifestyle causes diabetes can explain how it can best be managed.

Understanding Diabetes

We all use carbohydrates (sugar) for energy to live. Potatoes as well as chocolate bars are all converted into glucose (blood sugar) circulating in our blood stream. This sugar will be taken into the cells and "burned" to supply the energy to move a muscle or to think a thought or whatever it was that the cell is designed to do. But to get into a cell sugar must pass through a special sugar door in the cell's wall. These doors are how a cell tells the body it is hungry. A hungry cell will have thousands of these sugar doors all over its surface. Sugar by itself has no way to open these doors to get into the cell. Here is where insulin has its job.

Insulin

Imagine insulin as a little guy with two hands. With one hand he grabs the doorknob and opens one of these sugar doors and with the other hand he shoves a sugar through the door into the cell. Insulin opens the sugar doors.

Insulin comes from special cells in the pancreas called beta cells. These beta cells constantly taste your blood to see just how sweet it is. When they taste your sugar level rising after a meal they release more insulin into your blood. This insulin can then open more doors and put the extra sugar into the cells; thus, the amount of sugar left in the blood is brought back down to normal. This is how your body normally controls its blood sugar level.

Dealing with Raised Blood Sugar

Imagine sitting in an armchair, watching TV following a heavy meal. All of the calories you just ate are being absorbed into your blood. As your blood sugar level rises insulin is released.

This insulin goes around from cell to cell trying to open doors to get all of this sugar out of your blood and into your cells. But your leg muscle cells are still full of sugar from lunch! So they say to the insulin, "We are full and we aren't going for any exercise tonight so we don't need anymore sugar. Maybe you could take some to the finger muscle. He will be busy working the TV 'clicker.' But how much sugar can a finger muscle use? And so eventually all the muscle cells are stuffed and don't want any more sugar.

But how does a cell tell the body that it doesn't want any more sugar? It removes the doors from its surface! Now we have a problem. Where will the insulin take all of its extra sugar? Some cells can store extra sugar in the form of glycogen or fat. But day after day of no exercise while continuing to eat a high calorie diet will eventually overload these cells also. Not only do you get fat but even the fat cells are feeling stretched to their limit and don't want anymore calories. And now the problem gets worse. How does a fat cell tell you he is full and doesn't want anymore? He removes the doors from his surface too.

Now you have a serious problem. Where will the insulin take all of that extra sugar that you are eating? The answer is it has nowhere to go. It just backs up in your blood and your sugar level gets higher and higher. You go to your doctor and he does some tests and then he tells you that now you have diabetes.

Your doctor probably did something else for you that first

visit. He got out his prescription pad and wrote you a prescription for some tablets to lower your blood sugar. These tablets work by going to the beta cells in your pancreas and saying, "Make more insulin!" So the beta cells, whipped on by the medications, start to put out more insulin. All this extra insulin rushes around your body looking for a few last doors somewhere that they can force more sugar through.

After a time even these last few doors are removed. Your sugar levels continue to rise in spite of increasing doses of medication. Finally, one day your doctor says to you, "I guess the tablets are not working any more, so we are going to have to start you on insulin." However if you think carefully about how this disease has progressed to this point you will begin to see what the real problem is? Is it a lack of insulin or is it a lack of these sugar doors? The answer is there are not enough doors! The cells have removed all the doors because they aren't hungry anymore. So can you see that what we really need is not more insulin but more doors?

Your doctor can't prescribe a tablet or an injection for new doors for your cells. So how can we get more doors back on our cells? It is really quite simple. We have to make the cells hungry! A hungry cell will make thousands of doors all over its surface. How do we make a cell hungry? Exercise! Walk! Walk! Walk! Walk! This will help to reduce the risk of major complications as well.

The other half of the secret is that you have to learn to eat right so your body is not overloaded with calories. Research has shown that a wholefood diet allows people with diabetes to eat three meals a day and never go hungry and never count calories or exchanges again, whilst keeping their blood sugar under better control. This may seem surprising to some but the proof is seen in patients' success at the Weimar Institute in California, USA. Here clinicians have developed a programme using their own special version of this diet together with walking, all under close physician supervision and testing. This was the program that I followed and managed to successfully control diabetes, lose weight, reverse painful neuropathy and numbness in my fingers.

At The Weimar Institute they report 50% of people with **Type 2 diabetes** off all medication and insulin with a normal blood sugar in just 21 days. 80% of patients with neuropathy are pain free in just 17 days! Within a week of changing my lifestyle and eating habits, I was off all medication.

**Adapted from "How It Works -Diabetes Is Reversible!
By Dr Milton Teske
www.reversingdiabetes.org/?page=hiw**

A success story

On the 14th March 2002 I was told I had **Type 2 diabetes**, but like many people, I'd probably had it for years without realising it. I can't remember being told directly, but I surmised that this was the case through a series of questions the doctor asked.

The doctor on the end of the phone must have broken the news hundreds of times before. This time it was to me and I was unprepared.

He asked, "Is there diabetes in the family?"

"Yes," was my response "My father had it!"

In my mind, I reflected on my father, a slim man who had died some thirty years previous, quite mature in years, of what must have been something related to diabetes. I didn't really know, nor had I asked questions; however my nursing knowledge told me that this was possibly the case.

In a daze, I re-engaged with the doctor at the end of the phone.

"Do I have diabetes?" I asked.
The answer came back. " Your fasting blood sugar is 18 and your HbA1C is 11.8."

The latter didn't make much sense. I recalled that the normal blood sugar was somewhere between 3 and 6, but what was the HBA1C? I had never heard of it and I was too scared to ask. I later found out that this was quite a high reading, the norm for diabetics is between 4 and 6. But I will discuss this later.

All the symptoms that I had been experiencing over the previous four or so years collided in my mind. As a trained nurse, although I had not practised for years, the realisation of the diagnosis began to sink in, but I immediately started fighting back, not willing to accept the possible outcomes.

The symptoms had been real enough for a long time, but I had pushed them to the back if my mind. The most recent, blurred vision had been the most troublesome but I had put this down to reading a lot. The copious sweating, especially after eating meals and at nights, I had put down to 'the change', a thing most women had to put up with. Most of my friends were going through this, so why should I be any different? I took the advice of a friend, who had suggested eating small frequent meals. I ballooned from a neat size 12 to a rotund 20, bloated and ugly. Tingling feet, burning at nights, itching skin and a rash that would not go away, coupled with the need to purchase various creams to deal with the recurring skin problem.

All the books I read spoke of thirst, but I can only remember 3 days of this and the subsequent sweet- smelling urine as my kidneys could no longer cope with the raised levels of sugar that were being pumped through them. I was a diabetic. "Come and pick up a prescription," was the instruction that followed. Agreeing, I put the phone down.

Crushed and in despair, I later telephoned the surgery to make arrangements to collect the prescription and speak to the practice nurse if possible.

The receptionist managed to fit me in to see one of the nurses. As I waited, my mind went back to the medical wards of the 70s, when I was a junior nurse. All I remembered was measured calories, urine testing, insulin injections, and foot problems leading to amputations, kidney problems and eye problems. I did not want any of this. No Way! I was somewhat emotional by this point and could hardly hold back the tears.

Practice nurses see diabetics on a regular basis and to some extent were used to dealing with its management. But although anxious, I was also in rebellion. I did not want it, I did not invite it into my body and I needed a remedy, soon. A fight was on!

The nurse spoke to me reassuringly, telling me that things had changed since I trained in the 70s. Diabetics no longer had to weigh food, just eat a healthy diet. I thought I knew what a healthy diet was; at least I hoped so. I gratefully took home the leaflets that I was given and read them. However, the foods I loved were missing from their pages.

All my being, despite being broken, screamed rebellion to this invasion. I later told my husband, politely, not to mention it to anyone. Why? Fear and embarrassment had gripped me, yet in this silence, I had begun to search for loud answers.

I read books, articles anything that would show me a way out. As far as I was concerned, their pages spoke of doom and gloom. Why do writers feel compelled to tell sufferers of the negative side of the conditions, what to expect, over and over and over again? It was so depressing. Their pages offered little hope. Great! Yes! However, I am usually a positive person, keen to look for successes rather than failure. Their pages encouraged me to eat well and try to prevent hypos. List after list of instructions. The vague directions about eating healthily were the worse. This empty statement made me wonder what to eat!

Nevertheless, I began to eat three meals a day and within a 4-day span my medication was doubled to try to keep the blood sugar within a normal range. I was manic with worry as my urine measured 2%.

I later found out that I could buy a blood glucose monitor. I did. My readings were 12-14-16. I was determined never to let it get to 18 again, but at the time couldn't really get it under control.

Still my feet burned, especially at nights. My vision remained blurred, images distorted, fingertips numb and body cold. Nights, I dreaded them! There was no relief from the burning in my feet. Painkillers sometimes helped, but sleep was a luxury to be grabbed in the early hours of the morning.

I began to search for information. The Internet was intriguing. I found a web site and e-mailed someone asking for information to help with nutrition in **Type 2 diabetes.** They couldn't help. Still I searched. High carb! Low carb! Adkins diet! Still no help, but I kept searching; I knew the answer was out there somewhere. I just knew it.

The first week after diagnosis, my telephone rang. On the other end was a well known familiar voice. He spoke in strong, confident tones.

"Hi P, can you help me out this weekend, someone should be leading a seminar on stress but can't do it, can you?"

Hostility rose momentarily within me.

STRESS! Do you want to know STRESS," screamed my thoughts?"
A quiet voice came out of me. "Yes, I'll do it," I replied.

With blurred distorted vision, I searched the pages of a well-known book, trying to find a quick way to prepare for the subject area, when into mind dropped two words **reversing diabetes.**

The book, a Bible, had been purchased in 2001 at the IGOC Conference in London, England. Presented in its early pages is a list of topic areas with easy to find scriptures. The seminar I was asked to lead married the physical with the spiritual and so it was a natural choice for me.

As a Christian and former nurse, this experience has brought home the strong links between physical problems, spiritual values and belief systems. In times of need people rely more on their faith, something or someone that offers hope. I knew what I needed. Some of you reading, this, may begin to question what really happened, to others accepting it may be as natural as breathing. For those who have had similar experiences, it will be just something else that is extraordinary in our very ordinary lives.

With calm assurance, I rose from the settee and typed these two words into the web address on my computer. Logging on to the Internet was easy. I had done it several times over the past few days. Several web sites were displayed, but only one with the words reversing diabetes. It was in fact **www.reversingdiabetes.org**

I read its pages with urgency. The print was big and clear, useful when your vision is blurred. What I read gave me the hope that I was looking for. I rang and spoke to a health educator. He gave me simple, clear, concrete instructions, which allowed me a week later to discontinue medication and to begin to eat well, really well, healthily and more importantly, control my blood sugar safely. After three weeks the results were incredible! There were obvious changes in blood sugar level. Subsequent HbA1C readings showed marked improvements as demonstrated by the charts below.

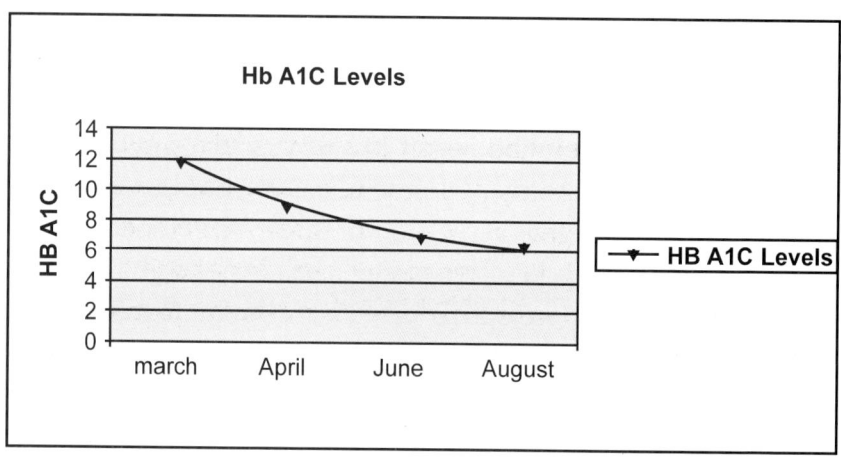

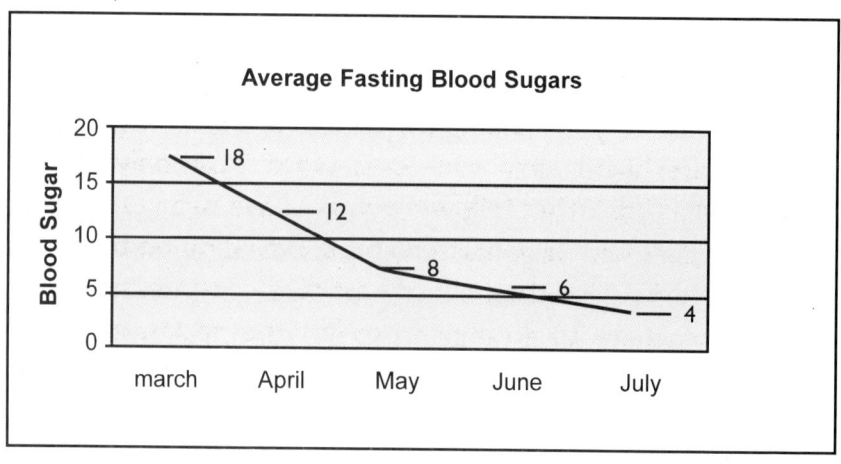

That was 15 months ago. I am now over 3 stones (42 lbs) lighter, wear a size 12-14 and have more vitality and energy than before and I am not anaemic. I have modified my lifestyle to fit in daily walks. In the beginning I walked after each meal. After a few weeks I began walking half an hour in the morning after breakfast and half an hour in the evening, still walking for 1 hr per day. I began to do this because I noticed that my blood sugar levels had began to show readings well below 10 mmol/L 2hrs after my main meal. Before I began to follow the principles taught at Weimar, sugar levels could be between 10-14 mmol/L. This really caused me to get excited. Nedley (1999) indicates that 30-45 minutes after eating a meal, the blood sugar rises to its maximum level and then returns gradually to a lower reading of between 5-7 mmol/L within a 2 hr time span and mine had begun to show similar characteristics. Blood sugar monitors are great for checking blood sugars accurately. If you haven't got one, I would suggest that you get one, as blood sugar readings will be more precise than urine testing only.

I know some of you reading this will have blood sugar readings that are higher than mine ever were. I can only suggest you try what I did. I am following what I have been taught and it worked for me. I have passed this information on to others and it is working for them. I now eat two or three meals per day. I don't have to go hungry. In fact the opposite is true. Once I started eating unprocessed, wholefoods I stayed fuller for longer. Drinking water between meals also gave me a sensation of fullness. If your blood sugar readings are above 10mmol/L 2 hours after eating a meal, just go for a 15 minute walk, if you can. When you return, take a rest and check your blood sugar reading. The results will surprise you. Your reading will be lower. It takes a lot of determination and motivation to do this, but it is worth it.

Often with high blood sugar come burning pains and/or pins and needles legs and feet. Should this happen, again go for a walk, there is a strong chance that the sensation will improve or disappear. Within 3 weeks of eating this way and following the walking plan, the numbness in my hands and feet began to disappear. More surprisingly, a numb white toe on my right foot became pink and the feeling returned. Previously, the soles of both feet (the right more so than the left) had been quite cyanosed, or blue in lay terms. Now I am happy to report that the circulation in both are much improved! The chiropodist recently complemented me on my feet, which was not the case when I first saw them back in March 2002. At that time they commented their coldness and compromised blood flow. It sounded so routine for them. Somehow I couldn't believe that they were referring to me, but they were. I took on board the information, but I refused to play the victim. I must also add that since changing my lifestyle sleep has also returned with real pleasure and fasting blood sugar readings have remained within a normal range 3.5 - 6.5 mmol/L.

Comments by Users of the Whole Plant Approach

Eating a whole plant food diet helped restore my blood pressure to normal...

My blood sugar was 25. After eating a whole plant food diet my early morning blood sugar was down to 8 in four days; now its down to 6 and I feel great...

My energy levels have increased...
My head feels a lot clearer - doesn't feel so thick...

I radically overhauled my diet and the first thing I noticed was that the strange feeling in my head disappeared...

My Hb A1C is coming down - it was 8...

My Hb A1C has come down from 11.8 to 6 in 4 months...

The tingling sensation in my legs and feet are gone

After 2 days, I didn't need my pills any more, my blood sugar was normal...

More energy... More vitality... More life... There is life after meat...equally as good or even better.

My fasting blood sugar used to be between 16 and 20, now it is between 5 and 7. I can sleep better at nights have lost 10lbs and can go up stairs more easily...My doctor is really pleased.

In March 2003 clinicians from The Weimar Institute carried out the first two day seminar on managing diabetes in the UK. During the weeks following the seminar, I was contacted by several participants who reportedly had become more active, were reducing their weight and reporting reduced symptoms of diabetes.

For example:
- Reduced sensation of pins and needles/burning in lower limbs

- Improved blood sugar control leading to decrease in insulin and tablet requirements

- Improved sleep pattern - less wakefulness

- Better blood pressure control

- Weight loss

- Reduced cholesterol level

- General feeling of well being

Diet and lifestyle

Background Information

Diabetes is a costly disease for those affected, their families, and health care systems. The disease process can lead to pain, anxiety, inconvenience, and impaired quality of life. It is the leading cause of blindness in adults in developed countries and the most common cause of amputation (WHO 2003). Those with diabetes are two to four times more likely to develop cardiovascular disease and strokes (WHO 2002). In the United Kingdom, around 5% of the total National Health Services (NHS) resources and up to 10% of hospitals' inpatient budgets are used for the care of people with diabetes (DoH 2002).

There is conclusive evidence that good control of blood glucose levels can substantially reduce the risk of developing complications and slow their progression (FAO & WHO 2003). The management of high blood pressure and raised blood lipids is equally important. Better control of these could contribute to a substantial improvement in quality of life (IDF 2003).

Evidence from Research

Crane and Sample (1994) tested the effect of a plant-based diet on patients with diabetic neuropathy in 21 adults enrolled in the 25-day Weimar Institute NEWSTART lifestyle program in California. They used a low fat, high fibre, total vegetarian diet (vegan), with exercise.

The diet included whole fruits and vegetables, whole grains, legumes, green leafy vegetables and mild herbs, and tubers. Nuts, olives, and avocados were allowed after weight was optimal for height; all but two participants were obese. 17 of the 21 had complete relief of painful neuropathy in 4 to 16 days. The remaining four had slight or partial relief. Five of the 21 no longer required insulin or hypoglycaemic drugs and those who did, required only on average 54% of the medication needed on entry to achieve the same or better blood sugar control.

Nicholson et al. (1999) conducted a small controlled pilot study of 11 men and women with type 2 diabetes. They were assigned either to a low fat total vegetarian (vegan) diet or a conventional low-fat diet. The vegan diet consisted of whole grains, fruit, vegetables, and legumes. All animal products, added oils, sugars and refined carbohydrates were excluded.

Fasting serum glucose, body weight, medication use, and blood pressure were assessed at intervals over 12 weeks. The results showed a 28% reduction for the experimental group in fasting blood glucose even in the absence of any exercise compared to a 12% decrease for the control group. Of the six subjects in the experimental group on oral hypoglycaemic drugs, medication use was discontinued for one and reduced for three. Insulin was reduced in the two patients in the experimental group on insulin, but in no patients in the control group. Vitamin B12 supplementation was recommended at the conclusion of the study for those continuing on the vegan diet.

In a small study, Barnard and colleagues (2003) examined the acceptability of a low fat, vegan diet in a controlled, 14-week trial involving 59 overweight American women. The women were randomly assigned to a low-fat, vegan, or National Cholesterol Education Program Step II diet. No differences between the groups on any acceptability measures were found suggesting that diet acceptability may not be a barrier to the use of low-fat vegan diets.

Pusey (1995) identified the need to include green bananas, cassava, breadfruit, sweet potato as examples of foods high in fibre, in the diet of African Caribbean people with type 2 diabetes.

The foods

I have used a range of foods, including those from the Caribbean. This exciting range provides a variety of colour, textures and appetising flavours that will stimulate your taste buds. It will help you manage **type two diabetes**, when used with a daily walking plan. The foods are neither boring nor repetitive. They are simple to use, economical and sustainable. To these foods are added vegetables and some fresh fruits to provide vitamins, minerals that the body need, and a daily dose of vitamin B 12. The diet is low in protein because a high protein diet puts a strain on the kidneys and most diabetics will need to avoid this (Nedley 1999). Plant based proteins are used instead of meat and dairy products, which are sources of animal protein as well as fat.

The recipes and advice in this book are based on foods from the Caribbean and principles taught to me during my stay at the Weimar Institute in California, USA in August 2002. I have used this advice to help others reduce high blood sugar safely, lose weight, have more energy and feel more in control. The foods are high in fibre, economical, simple and easy to prepare, and burst with flavour on your tongue. These are known as whole plant foods.

These principles are useful for managing;

- Obesity

- Overweight

- Hypertension

- Coronary Heart Disease

- Raised Cholesterol

A whole plant food diet is based on complex carbohydrates such as whole grain cereals - wheat, oats, rice, barley, millet, etc, potatoes, whole grain rice, beans, lentils, and more. The diet provides the proper fuel for the diabetic. Whole plant foods are unprocessed and unrefined grains, vegetables, fruits and nuts. These are high fibre foods and offer a number of benefits to people with Type two diabetes.
www.weimar.org.

These principles are supported by research evidence and have for more than 20 years successfully managed patients with diabetes, high blood pressure, coronary artery disease, arteriosclerosis and arthritis (Nedley 1999). I learned first hand of the success that can be gained through changes in diet and following an exercise programme. During my stay I found that not only were diabetics reducing their need for tablets and insulin, those with high blood pressure and cholesterol saw their level fall within a few days of eating a whole plant food diet and following an exercise plan of walking daily. Details are outlined on pages 32 and 33. To help you monitor your progress daily walking diaries have been included for you to complete. (See pages 34-37).

The Recipes

The recipes suggested are low in fat, but are not fat free as they contain plant-based fatty acids. Therefore you will avoid all of the harmful saturated fats and cholesterol found in animal products. Refined, processed foods are also excluded, as these are not wholefoods.

Stocking up with Wholefoods

A range of food items can be found in Asian food stores, health food shops and local supermarkets like Sainsbury and Tesco.

Having made the decision to eat more healthily, it is essential to make changes to what we would normally choose to have in the kitchen cupboard, fridge and freezer. First of all remove all the foods that you no longer want to use from the kitchen. If the rest of the family is not eating like you, have a separate cupboard for your foodstuff. Here are some suggestions for achieving easy meal preparation.

Kitchen cupboard should include:
· Tinned foods such as beans, tomatoes, sugar free pasta sauce, tomato puree / sauce, salsa

· Wholewheat pasta, corn, whole grain rice, wholewheat cous cous and other grains

· Potatoes, Yam, Sweet Potatoes, Casava, Breadfruit, Dasheen

· Dried legumes, e.g. kidney beans, butter beans, chickpeas, black-eyed beans and lentils

· Whole grain breakfast cereals such as weetabix, shredded wheat, cornmeal bran flakes, rolled oats, oatmeal and bulgar wheat

· Dried fruits such as dates, raisins and pineapples

· Packaged milk such as rice, oats and soya

· A variety of nuts especially almonds and cashews, sunflower, pumpkin and sesame seeds

· Low salt vegetarian stock cubes and seasonings

· Garlic and onion powder

· Various herbs such as thyme, sage and parsley etc.

In the freezer:
· Mixed vegetables - a wide range

- Fruit juices

- Berries for cooking

- Wholewheat bread

In the fridge:
- Fresh fruit and vegetables

- Various home-made spreads - see section an the end of this book e.g. orange cashew spread.

- Fresh tofu

- Soya sauce

Making Walking a Part of Your Daily Routine

Being told that your are a **Type 2 diabetic** is likely to be difficult to come to terms with. Most diabetics have been told that, "You are a diabetic. You will always be a diabetic. You can try to control it with diet, medications or insulin but you cannot reverse it or cure it. Once you have diabetes you will always have diabetes." From experience I have found that a change in the foods we eat can, together with a daily exercise plan, help to maintain glucose levels, lose weight, make you feel more energetic and in control of rather than being controlled by diabetes.

To some of you reading this, the thought of walking a few metres may be problematic. Maybe walking has not been a part of your routine for some time. However, it has been found that walking, when used in combination with a whole plant food diet will help to control your blood sugar safely and may help in reducing the need for tablets or insulin (Crane and Sample 1994). Other forms of exercise will also help, but walking is an economical and better option for most people.

Begin slowly, have a routine and plan your day including your meals. Have a reason for walking, for example, to buy a newspaper, post a letter, or visit a friend. Once you begin to gain confidence, you will notice that walking is more enjoyable than you first thought. Gradually increase your walking time to thirty minutes in the morning, repeated in the evening. Eventually you will be walking 2-3 miles per day without realising this. Try walking after your morning and evening meals as this will help to reduce the steep rise in blood sugar levels, often seen in diabetes.

What about Footwear?

Make sure that you wear comfortable footwear, sturdy and suitable for people with diabetes. If in doubt ask a podiatrist for advice on safe walking footwear for diabetics. Remember to dress according to the weather and not the season. Research evidence has also shown that the ideas suggested here can help diabetics reduce weight, painful neuropathy and other complications (Crane and Sample 1994).

Walking Helps To:

· Improve your circulation

· Increase muscle activity and assist the body in using up excess blood glucose, thereby reducing blood glucose levels and insulin resistance

· Provide exercise and increase muscle tone

· Assist in improving the body's immune response

Some Suggestions when Considering Walking:

· If you are unable to get out, walk around the house. It is good exercise. I sometimes walk around when I'm on the phone.

· If you are a little unsteady on your feet or are not happy to walk by yourself, ask someone to walk with you.

· Walk with a friend or form a walking club.

· Instead of taking the bus or the car why not walk half the journey

· Map out some local routes with the car. For example ½ mile, 1 mile, 1½ miles, 2 miles etc. This helps you to know how far you are walking.

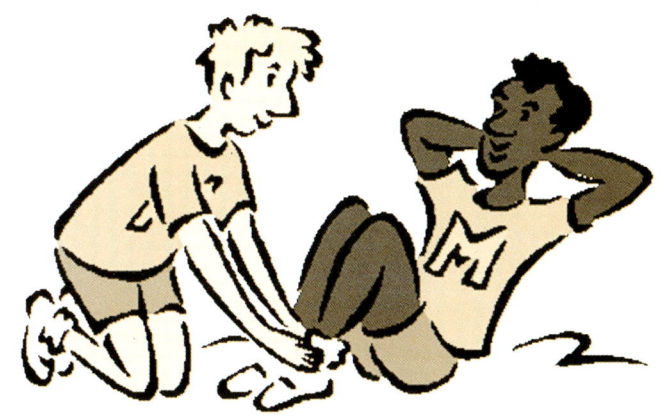

Looking after Your Feet:

· Wash feet daily in lukewarm water using a mild soap.

· Avoid soaking your feet as this dries the skin, which can lead to cracks and fissures that may become easily infected.

· After bathing, dry using a soft towel, especially between the toes.

· If your skin is dry, use a little cream or lotion to moisture the skin.

· If the skin is too moist, use powder to dry it a little.

· Inspect your feet daily for cracks in the skin, cuts, blister, ingrown toenails, excessive calluses or corns and "hot" spots that may be red, or the beginning of an infection. Report these to your health care provider-doctor, nurse or podiatrist.

· Avoid cutting your own nails; filing is better. Use an emery board; file straight across do not shape the nails like a fingernail, except to round off sharp corners.

· Use warm blankets or socks to keep your feet warm. Never use a heating pad or hot water bottle. Keep your feet warm; do not make them warm.

· Before putting on shoes turn them upside down and shake them to empty out anything that may have fallen inside. Feel for lumpiness of any kind, torn lining, nails or anything coming through the sole. Take a look inside to see if anything is wrong with the shoe.

· Keep your shoes on. **Do not** go bare footed.

· Elevate your feet to the level with your hips, while sitting, once or twice per day to aid circulation.

· No high heels! Wear as low a heel as you can. Flat heels are preferred. Heels of any height can throw your feet off balance and produce pressure where your foot was not meant to have pressure, such as the 'ball' of the foot.

· Wear well fitting shoes. There must be room for the toes to move a little and the heel must be snug enough to keep from rubbing the heel.

· Try shoes on and walk around the store enough so that you can tell if they fit your foot. They should be soft enough to be comfortable and strong enough to give support. Wear shoes for comfort and not for fashion.

Characteristics of Good Socks

· The foot should fit in the sock smoothly so as not to cause wrinkles inside the shoe. Socks that move or roll around and get lumpy should not be worn.

· The ankle and leg part of the sock should be smooth and not too tight. If it causes a line on your leg that shows up when the sock comes off, they are too tight. Take some scissors and clip a small notch in the very top of the sock to get rid of this.

· No darns, no seams, no lumps and wrinkles inside the sock. Invert the socks if necessary so that seams are worn on the outside.

How to Maximise Blood Sugar Control - Byers Model
adapted from the Newstart Lifestyle Programme

Activity	Value of activity
It is **important** to keep in regular contact with your doctor and specialist nurse.	To monitor changes in your health and to adjust your medications according to the changes that are occuring.
Walk for at least 15 minutes immediately after each meal. If this is not possible aim to walk at least 30 mins both after breakfast and evening meal.	To reduce the immediate rise in blood sugar. As soon as you eat the blood sugar starts to rise, walking immediately after eating keeps the blood sugar from going as high.
Walk a total of at least 60 minutes each day	Exercise decreases insulin resistance and helps the body use the insulin that is available.
2 - 3 meals a day and NO snacking	Snacking raises the blood sugar and may keep it unnecessarily high.
Up to 2 servings of fruit for breakfast, none after breakfast (up to ½ a banana is one serving) Daily vitamin B12	Too much fruit may raise the blood sugar excessively. You have the whole day to use the extra carbohydrates that will come with the fruit. **Do not** eat 5 pieces of fruit a day, 2 are enough.

Activity	Value of activity
No juices - fruit or vegetable unless hypoglycaemic	Hypoglycaemia is when the blood sugar is <3.3 mmol/L.
Whole plant foods eaten whole (see page 25 and recipe section). No dairy products, use soya products instead.	Delays the absorption of carbohydrates and calories and thus your blood sugar will not rise as rapidly.
No dried / cooked fruit	Concentrated food raises the sugar too rapidly, good if you are hypoglycaemic.
Eat salads first	Delays the absorption of calories and blood sugar will go up more slowly.
Eat slowly	Food absorbed more slowly and blood sugar will not increase as rapidly.
Drink 2½ -3 litres water daily, not at mealtime. Drink 2 full glasses on waking.	Better hydration, more efficient operation of our body.
Eliminate caffinated beverages	Caffeine is a stimulant and will tend to aggravate stress. Those who use stress management have been shown to have lower blood sugars.

Daily walking Diary

week 1					weight
day	blood glucose a.m	time walked after breakfast	blood glucose p.m	time walked after evening meal	
1					
2					
3					
4					
5					
6					
7					

Daily walking Diary

week 2   weight

day	blood glucose a.m	time walked after breakfast	blood glucose p.m	time walked after evening meal
1				
2				
3				
4				
5				
6				
7				

Daily walking Diary

week 3   weight

day	blood glucose a.m	time walked after breakfast	blood glucose p.m	time walked after evening meal
1				
2				
3				
4				
5				
6				
7				

Daily walking Diary

week **4**   weight

day	blood glucose a.m	time walked after breakfast	blood glucose p.m	time walked after evening meal
1				
2				
3				
4				
5				
6				
7				

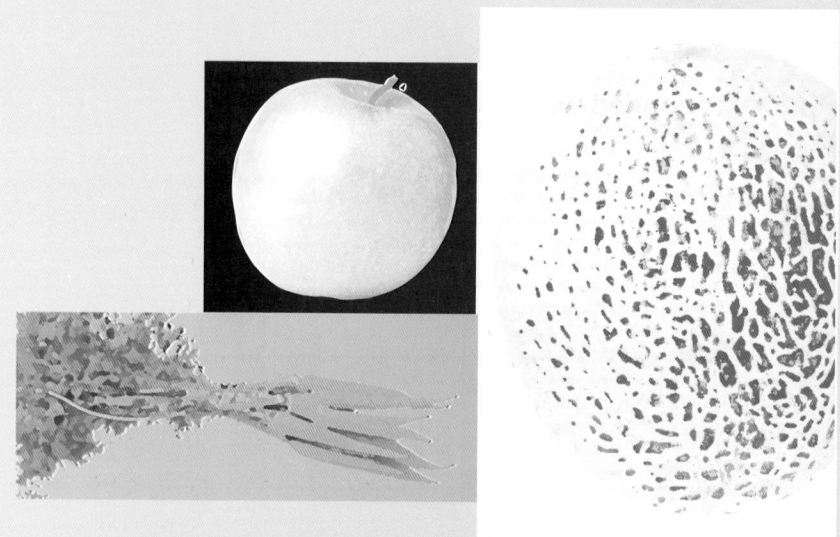

Recipes
Whole plant Foods

Main Courses

* These recipes have been used with the kind permission of the Weimar Institute California USA

Chickpea Burgers

1 tin cooked chickpeas
1 large onion chopped
1 cup uncooked rolled oats
1 tablespoon soy sauce
1 cup finely chopped walnuts
$\frac{1}{2}$ cup water
$\frac{1}{2}$ teaspoon salt and $\frac{1}{2}$ teaspoon garlic powder
$\frac{1}{4}$ cup dried parsley
$\frac{1}{2}$ teaspoon sage

Blend chickpeas with some of the water till smooth. Repeat with onion and walnuts and add both mixtures to mixing bowl. Add remaining ingredients and mix well. Let stand for up to $\frac{1}{2}$ hour or refrigerate for several hours. Shape into burgers and bake in the oven gas mark 6 for 15 -20 mins - makes 15 to 20 burgers. Burgers freeze well. (Chickpeas can be substituted with other beans)

Parsnip Burgers

1 cup cooked kidney beans
1 cup cooked whole grain rice
$\frac{1}{4}$ cup chopped cashew nuts
2 parsnips - peeled, cooked and mashed - keep broth
1 cup broth from parsnips
2 tablespoons oats
1 teaspoon soy sauce
1 teaspoon garlic
1 teaspoon onion seasoning

1 teaspoon garlic
1 teaspoon onion seasoning
1 teaspoon thyme
1 onion chopped
½ red pepper chopped

Process all ingredients together in a blender until smooth. Shape into burgers or use a serving spoon to place mixture on well-greased baking tray. Bake on gas mark 4 for 20 mins turning once. Great for buns with soya cheese and salad - Soya cheese is available from health food shops.

Super Burger

125g tofu mashed
1 cup walnuts
1 cup oats
1 medium onion chopped
1 teaspoon garlic paste
½ cup water
1 teaspoon thyme
1 teaspoon sage
1 teaspoon vegan powder

Mash tofu with a fork. Add all other ingredients except water - mix well. Add water. Leave to stand for ½ hour. Use an ice-cream scoop to shape into mounds. Place mounds on lightly greased baking tray. Press mound flat with the back of a desert spoon. Bake at gas mark 6 for 30 mins - turning once. Serve in wholewheat pitta bread filled with salad.

Mixed Bean Stew with Plantain Dumpling

1 cup red kidney beans
1 cup butter beans
1 cup pinto beans (tinned beans can be used - rinse to reduce salt content or better still buy organic, they are usually salt free)
2 carrots chopped
1x 250g tin of tomatoes chopped
1 green pepper chopped
1 cup wholewheat flour
¼ ripened plantain grated
½ teaspoon salt
1 teaspoon garlic powder
1 teaspoon paprika
1 teaspoon onion powder
1 teaspoon thyme
2 tablespoons cornflour

If using dried beans pre-soak these over night. Pour off water. Add 1 litre of water, bring to the boil and simmer until tender - 45-60 mins. Place wholewheat flour in a bowl. Add grated plantain and a little salt. Mix to firm dough with a little water - add more flour if necessary. Form into tiny finger shapes - add to bean mixture. Add more water to bean mixture if necessary. Bring mixture to the boil - add other ingredients - simmer for 20-25 mins. Mix cornflour to paste with a little water, add to mixture. Add more seasoning to taste. Simmer for 5 mins - serve hot with boiled whole grain rice, jacket potatoes or yam and a range of hot and cold vegetables.

* Eggplant Casserole

1 small eggplant, thinly sliced
1 onion, thinly sliced
1 red pepper, sliced
250g (1 lb) firm tofu
1 large can crushed tomatoes
1 small can tomato paste

Mash tofu fine with a fork. Add 1 tablespoon basil, $1/2$ teaspoon salt, and 1 teaspoon onion powder & blend well. Prepare a 9x12 inch dish. Layer with half the sliced eggplant, half the onions, half the pepper and half the tofu. Repeat. Mix tomato paste with crushed tomatoes (add a little water - just enough for rinsing cans). Pour tomato mixture over top of casserole. Bake for an hour at gas mark 6, covered with foil.

Walnut a la King - Meatballs

2 cups finely ground walnuts
1 cup cooked bulgar wheat
1 $1/2$ cups of boiling water
$1/2$ cup wholewheat bread crumbs
1 med. onion finely chopped
2 tablespoons wholewheat flour
1 tablespoon soy sauce
2 cloves garlic finely chopped
1 teaspoon parsley

To prepare bulgar wheat

Add boiled water to bulgar wheat - cover and leave to stand for 10 mins. Place all other ingredients in a bowl. Drain off excess water off bulgar wheat by placing it in a sieve. Add 1 cup of bulgar wheat to other ingredients. Mix ingredients gently with a fork - do not press together. To obtain meat ball shape use an ice cream server to scoop mixture from the bowl. Place meatballs on lightly greased baking tray- bake on gas mark 5 for 20-25 mins. Serve with Salsa Dip, see page 97.

Corny Wheat

1 cup frozen corn
1 cup bulgar wheat
2 ½ cups boiling water
1 teaspoon salt
2 sprigs spring onions chopped
1 teaspoon sage
1 teaspoon thyme

Place bulgar wheat in a bowl and add 1 cup boiling water. Add all other ingredients except corn - cover and leave to stand for 10 mins. Drain liquid from corn. Place remaining cup of water in a small pan. Add corn and bring to the boil. Simmer for 2-3 mins and drain. Add to bulgar wheat mixture and stir until corn is dispersed. Add remaining ½ cup of water and leave to cook slowly on a low heat for 10-15 mins. Serve immediately.

Cous Cous

1 cup cous cous
1 cup of boiling water
2 sprigs spring onion chopped
1 teaspoon thyme
½ teaspoon sea salt
A few black olives chopped
4 cherry tomatoes chopped
½ red or green pepper chopped

Place cous cous in a bowl. Add water and cover for 5 mins - add remaining ingredients - stir with a fork and serve. For variation, add a few herbs, red and or green peppers and beans of choice.

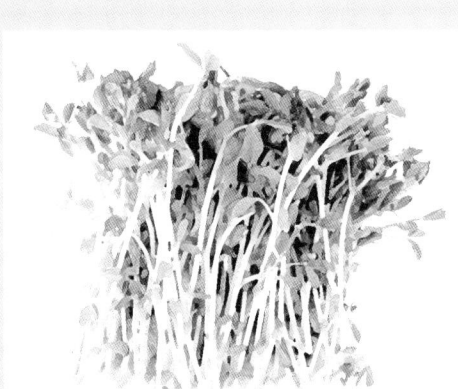
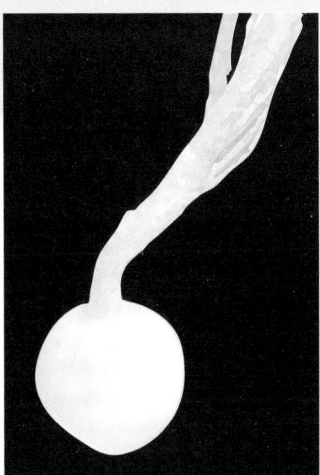

Cooking with Tofu

Tofu is a complete vegetable protein food made in a simple process from soya bean, and is nutritious. It is low in fat and a good source of protein and can be used in a variety of dishes. A few examples are given here.

* Scrambled Tofu

1x 250g pack firm tofu
1 medium onion
1 large tomato
½ medium green pepper
Salt, garlic powder and basil - season to taste
¼ to ½ teaspoon turmeric (yellow)

Chop the onions and green pepper and sauté in a small amount of olive oil. Add the tofu and mash to a scrambled egg consistency. Add turmeric (for colour) and season with salt garlic powder and basil to taste. Cut the tomato into small chunks and add last. Cook a little more. Good scrambled egg substitute. also good as a breakfast dish.

Saucy Tofu

1x 250g pack tofu
1 teaspoon sage
1 teaspoon thyme
2 teaspoons vegetable seasoning
1 teaspoon parsley
1 teaspoon onion powder
1 teaspoon garlic powder or paste
2 tablespoons cornflour
1½ - 2 cups water
A little olive oil

Place vegetable seasoning on a plate. Cut tofu into strips. Dip tofu strips individually into vegetable seasoning. Grease frying pan - heat gently. Place tofu in heated greased frying pan. Brown 1-2 mins each side.

In a small bowl place 3 tablespoons tomato paste and water. Add 1 teaspoon sage, 1 teaspoon parsley, 1 teaspoon onion powder and 1 teaspoon garlic powder or paste. Mix well and pour over tofu. Mix cornflour in a little water and add to mixture. Stir until thickens. Add salt to taste. Simmer for 3-5 mins. Serve with Pasta. For variation - cooked beans, mixed vegetables or cooked aubergines can be added to the mixture.

Tofu and Aubergine Casserole

2 x 250g packet tofu cut into chunks
3 tomatoes chopped finely
1 aubergine cut in thin slices
2 tablespoons tomato puree
1 teaspoon vegan bouillon powder (available from Tesco)
1 onion chopped
½ teaspoon basil
2 cups of boiling water
2 teaspoons garlic powder
1 tablespoon soy sauce
1 tablespoons cornflour

Toss tofu in bouillon powder. Leave to stand for ½ hr or overnight in a fridge. Place tofu on lightly greased tray and bake in hot oven gas mark 6 for 25 mins - until brown. In a wok place 1 cup water and chopped onions, simmer until onions are tender, add tomatoes and simmer for 2-3 mins. Add remaining ingredients - except basil - bring to the boil and simmer for 5 mins - add tofu - bring to the boil and simmer for 7-10 mins or until aubergine is tender. Mix cornflour in a little water and add to mixture and stir until it thickens slightly. Add basil and simmer for 2-3 mins. Serve on a bed of whole grain rice, pasta or cous cous and a range of hot and cold vegetables.

Tofu Megadrive

3 cups water
1 x 250g block of tofu cut into chunks
3 sprigs of spring onions chopped finely
1 vegetable stock cube
1 onion chopped
1 tablespoon vegetable mix
2 tablespoons parsley chopped
1 teaspoon onion powder
1 teaspoon garlic powder
1 small tin tomatoes chopped
1 small tin chick peas

Prepare tofu as on previous page. Place 1 cup of water in a frying pan. Add chopped onion. Simmer for 3 mins until tender. Add chopped tomatoes simmer for a further 2 minutes. Add remaining ingredients except tofu and cornflour and parsley. Be sure to add remaining water and crumble stock cube into mixture - stir well. Bring to the boil and simmer until courgettes are cooked. Add tofu and parsley. Mix cornflour in a little water, add to mixture, cook for a further 3 mins. Serve on a bed of rice. Also good with pasta, cous cous and baked potatoes.

Tofu A La King

1 x 250g tofu cut into eight strips
2 cups water
1/4 cup cashews
2 tablespoons soy sauce
1 teaspoon garlic powder, 1 teaspoon onion powder
2/3 large tomatoes chopped
1 medium onion chopped
1 red sweet pepper, 1 green pepper - chopped
2 cups water
1 teaspoon basil
1 teaspoon thyme
1/2 teaspoon bouillon powder (available from Tesco)
1-2 tablespoons wholewheat flour

Place chunks of tofu in a small bowl. Mix soy sauce, onion powder and garlic powder together. Pour mixture over tofu - cover and leave to marinade over night preferably or stand for 1/2 an hour. Place blocks of tofu on lightly greased baking tray. Bake for 25 mins gas mark 6.

In a frying pan, add 1 cup water and chopped onions. Cook until tender. Add cashews. Add other ingredients. Bring to the boil and simmer for 3-5 mins. Add herbs. Mix wholewheat flour in a little water and add to mixture in pan. Simmer for a while longer. Add tofu to mixture, stir and serve with pasta and a range of vegetables.

Rainbow Tofu Stir Fry

A little olive oil to grease wok
1 x 250g block tofu
½ cup water
1 onion finely chopped
4 cups cold cooked whole grain rice - (cooked from previous day preferably)
1 red pepper
1 teaspoon garlic paste
1 table spoon soy sauce
1 teaspoon onion granule
1 cup frozen mixed vegetable

Cut tofu into small cubes. Grease wok and heat, add tofu and brown for 2 mins each side. Remove tofu from wok. Add water to wok, chopped onion, mixed vegetable, garlic, onion granules, soy sauce and red pepper. Cook on a high heat until water almost gone. Add rice and heat through thoroughly 3-4 mins on a medium heat. Add tofu, stir and serve with salad.

Sweet and Sour Tofu

1 packet (250g) tofu
2 cups water
1 teaspoon garlic powder
1 teaspoon onion powder
1 large tin tomatoes chopped
1 medium onion chopped
1 red sweet pepper and 1 green pepper - chopped

Juice of 1 lemon
1 tablespoon honey
1 tablespoon soy sauce
1 small tin pineapple chunks
1 teaspoon basil and 1 teaspoon thyme
½ teaspoon bouillon powder
1-2 tablespoons cornflour

Cut tofu into cubes. Place bouillon powder on a small plate. Toss tofu gently in mixture. Place blocks of tofu on lightly greased baking tray. Bake for 25 mins gas mark 6, until golden brown.

To make sweet and sour sauce

Place 1 cup of water in a frying pan. Add chopped onion - sauté until tender. Add chopped tomatoes - simmer for 2 mins - crushing as you stir. Add chopped pepper, pineapple, and honey and lemon juice. Add remaining water. Mix cornflour in a little water and add to mixture. Cook for further 2 mins. Add tofu - simmer for 1 minute. Add basil and thyme. Serve on bed of rice - with a range of cooked and raw vegetables.

Tofu Asian Charm

1 pack (250g) tofu cut into chunks (about 16)
¼ cup whole cashew nuts
1 tablespoon soy sauce
1 teaspoon garlic powder
1 teaspoon onion powder
2/3 large tomatoes chopped
1 medium onion chopped
1 red sweet pepper, 1 green pepper - chopped
2 cups water
1 teaspoon basil
1 teaspoon cumin
1 teaspoon thyme
½ -1 teaspoon bouillon powder
1½ -2 tablespoons wholewheat flour

Place blocks of tofu in a small bowl. Mix soy sauce, onion powder and garlic powder together. Pour mixture over tofu - cover and leave to marinade over night preferably or stand for ½ an hour. Place blocks of tofu on lightly greased baking tray. Bake for 25 mins gas mark 6 until lightly brown.

To make sauce

Place 1 cup of water in a frying pan. Add chopped onion - sauté until tender. Add tomatoes - simmer for two minutes - crushing as you stir. Add chopped pepper, bouillon powder, cashews and remaining water. When tender sprinkle in wholewheat flour. Cook for further 2 mins. Put tofu in the mixture - simmer for 1 min. Add basil and thyme. Add tofu - serve on bed of whole grain rice with a range of vegetables.

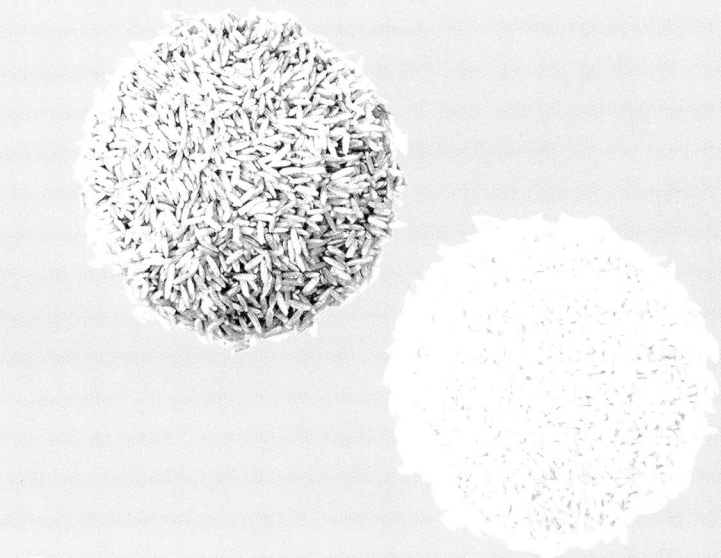

Cooking with Whole Grain Rice

Boiled whole grain rice

2 cups of whole grain rice
4 cups of water,
½ teaspoon salt

Bring water to the boil. Add rice and salt. Allow to boil for 5 minutes. Lower heat. Cover firmly and simmer gently for 35-40 mins.

Savoury Rice

4 cups water
2 cups rice
1 tomato
2 cloves garlic - crushed
1½ teaspoons vegan bouillon powder (available from Tesco)
1 medium onion chopped
1 red capsicum - cut into strips
½ teaspoon onion powder, ½ teaspoon paprika

Place water in pan. Add rice - bring to the boil. Boil vigorously for 5 mins. Add remaining ingredients. Stir gently with a fork. Simmer for 35-40 mins over low heat until all water absorbed. Serve hot with salad, cooked vegetables and bean salad.

Caribbean Rice

4 cups water
2 cups whole grain rice
½ cup unsweetened desiccated coconut
1 cup cooked kidney beans

1 clove garlic
½ teaspoon vegan bouillon powder
1 teaspoon sweet basil
medium onion chopped
½ teaspoon onion powder, ½ teaspoon paprika

Bring water to the boil, add rice - boil vigorously for 5 mins in covered pan. Add chopped onions and other ingredients. Bring to the boil again; stir gently with a fork. Cook on a low heat for 35-40 mins. Serve hot with salad and cooked vegetables. Kidney beans can be substituted with black-eyed beans, pinto beans etc, but remember to cook these before adding to the rice.

Melody Rice

4 cups water
1 cup whole grain rice
2 cups cooked chickpeas - tinned
2 cloves garlic chopped
1 cup frozen green peas
½ - 1 teaspoon bouillon powder
1 red and 1 green pepper cut into strips
2 medium onions chopped
½ - 1 teaspoon onion powder
1 teaspoon paprika

Bring water to the boil, add rice - boil vigorously for 5 mins in covered pan. Add other ingredients. Bring to the boil again; stir gently with a fork. Cook on a low heat for 35 - 40 mins. Serve hot with salad and cooked vegetables.

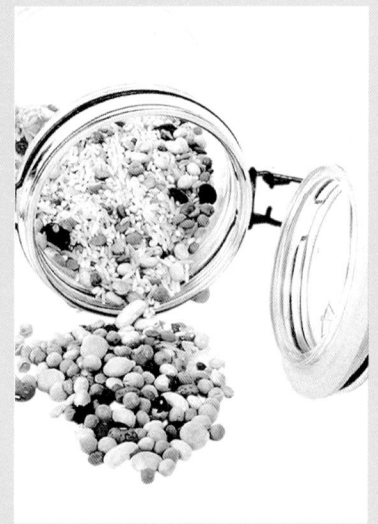

Cooking with Beans

Tips on cooking Beans

Most beans will need soaking over night in cold water except black-eyed beans. These do not need lengthy soaking and take about 1 hour to cook. Most other beans e.g. kidney beans, butter beans, and chickpeas do and cooking times vary from between 1½ to 2 hours, or until tender. To cook beans, drain away the water that they have been soaking in, add fresh water, bring to the boil for ten minutes, reduce the heat and simmer until beans are tender. If you need to top up with water use hot boiled water from a kettle. Add seasonings after the beans are tender as adding these before may interfere with the tendering process.

Three Bean Salad

1 cup each of three cooked beans
e.g. kidney, pinto, black-eyed or butter beans
1/4 - 1/2 teaspoon each parsley, sage, rosemary and thyme 1
1 tablespoon lemon juice (optional)
Salt to taste
Place all ingredients in a bowl - mix well and serve with mix green salad.

Green Bean Salad

250g frozen green beans
240g tin of red kidney beans
1 teaspoon vegan bouillon powder (optional) available from Tesco
1 cup water

Bring water to boil. Add green beans - bring to boil again. Cover and simmer until tender - water may have evaporated, if not, drain. Add drained kidney beans. Sprinkle with vegan bouillon powder - stir and serve.

Cashew and Onion salad

1/2 cup water
4 sprigs of spring onion chopped
1 onion chopped
1/2 red pepper sliced
1/2 green pepper sliced
2 cups unsalted cashews
2 tablespoons tomato puree in a further 1/2 cup of water

1 teaspoon vegan bouillon powder
1 teaspoon parsley
Juice of ½ lemon

Place ½ cup of water in a saucepan and add all onions. Add cashews and heat through thoroughly stirring all the time. Add tomato paste in water. Add all other ingredients. Stir continually. Heat thoroughly and serve hot.

Bean and Vege Concert

4 cups water
1 x 250g tin red kidney or pinto beans - drained
1 medium onion sliced finely
1 green pepper, finely chopped
3 tablespoons tomato puree
1 teaspoon garlic paste
1 x 450gm packet Realeat vege-mince (available from Tesco)
1 tablespoon soy sauce
Pinch of salt
1 tablespoon wholewheat flour
1 tablespoon sesame seeds (optional)
A pinch of thyme

Place ½ cup water in a wok. Add onion, tomato puree, garlic paste and pepper. Bring to the boil and simmer for 5 mins, until onions cooked. Add remaining water and bring to the boil. Add vege-mince and beans - bring to the boil again. Turn heat low and simmer for 10 -15 mins. Sprinkle with 1 tablespoon wholewheat flour and stir gently - cook a little longer. Add thyme and sesame seeds, stir and serve on a bed of whole grain rice, Serve with side salad and cooked vegetables. (Also goes well with baked potatoes, pasta or sweet potatoes).

Butter Bean Casserole

1 x 250g tin of organic butter beans
2 carrots - peeled and chopped
1 medium onion chopped
1 tablespoon soy sauce
1-2 tablespoons breadcrumbs
1 tablespoon parsley
1 teaspoon each of garlic, thyme, basil

Place butter bean and liquid in a pan. Add chopped carrots and finely chopped onion. Bring to the boil - simmer until carrots are cooked. Thicken with a little cornflour or wholemeal breadcrumbs. Add the remaining ingredients. Simmer for additional 2-3 mins. Serve with rice / baked potatoes / yam etc plus a range of vegetables.

Broccoli and Butter Beans

500g broccoli
2 cups water
1 x 200g tin chopped tomatoes
1 x 400g tin butter beans
1 onion chopped

½ vegetable stock cube - optional
1 teaspoon rosemary - optional
1 teaspoon parsley
Juice of ½ a lemon
1 tablespoon soy sauce
2 tablespoons cornflour - mixed in a little water

Place 1 cup of water in a pan. Dissolve stock cube in it. Add onions and garlic. Cook until tender. Add tomatoes and butter beans. Bring mixture to the boil. Wash broccoli and cut florets in half if large and add to mixture in pan Simmer for 10 mins - or until tender. Add remaining ingredients except cornflour - stir gently. Mix cornflour in a little water and add to mixture - bring to the boil. Stir gently and serve. Good with whole grain rice or filling for jacket potatoes on a bed of whole grain rice.

Cassava, Bean and Plantain Casserole

½ cup each of the following black-eyed, kidney, chickpeas and pinto beans.
3 cloves garlic - crushed
3 medium carrots chopped (about 250g, ½ lb)
500g (1lb) cassava
1 green plantain
1 red pepper - chopped
3 sprigs of spring onion- chopped
1 large onion chopped
2-3 cups boiling water
1 vegetable stock cube

1 teaspoon each of sage, oregano, and thyme
1 teaspoon onion granules
1 teaspoon paprika
Salt to taste
2 tablespoons cornflour
A dash of soy sauce (optional)

Wash, and cover beans with water. Leave to soak over night. Drain away water and place beans in a medium sized saucepan. Cover with water. Bring to the boil and leave to simmer for 1 - 1½ hrs or until all beans are tender. Chop all onions, carrots, and red pepper into small pieces and add to the saucepan. Peel cassava and green plantain, cut into 1 inch pieces and place in pot. Cover with boiling water so that all vegetables are just covered - (2 cups). Bring to the boil, reduce heat and simmer until all vegetables are tender. Mix cornflour in a little water and add to mixture. Stir well. Add remaining ingredients and salt to taste. Serve with a range of cooked vegetables.

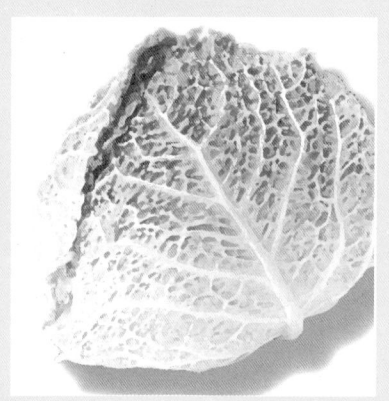
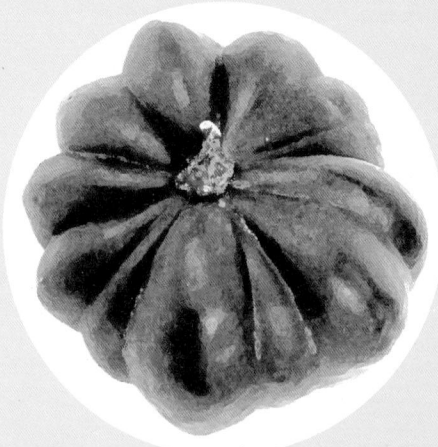

Cooking with a Range of Vegetables

Lentil and Vegetable Soup

½ cup lentils
1 litre water
2 leeks - cut thinly
1 stock cube
2 medium sized carrots chopped
1 medium sized parsnip chopped
1 teaspoon garlic paste
1 teaspoon mixed herb
1 medium sized onion chopped
1 sprig of spring onion

Bring water to the boil. Add lentils, bring to the boil and simmer for 10 minutes. Add remaining ingredients except for herbs. Bring to the boil and simmer for 10 mins. Blend with a hand processor. Add mixed herbs. Serve.

Butter bean and Leek Soup

1 litre water
1 tin organic butter beans drained (250g)
1 medium onion finely chopped
3 cloves of garlic chopped
2 leeks chopped
1 organic stock cube
1 teaspoon dried basil

Bring water to boil and add chopped leeks, garlic and stock cube. Cook until tender. Add butter beans, bring to the boil again. Remove from stove and blend with hand blender.

Add very finely chopped onion simmer for 2 mins. Add basil - stir and serve.

Mixed Vegetable Soup

1 sliced pumpkin - cut into small piece
½ cup lentils
1 litre water
1 stock cube
1 medium sized carrot chopped
1 medium sized parsnip chopped
3 cloves garlic
1 teaspoon mixed herbs
1 medium sized onion chopped
2 sprigs of spring onion

Bring water to the boil Add lentils, bring to the boil and simmer for 10 mins. Add remaining ingredients except for herbs. Bring to the boil and simmer for 10 mins. Blend with a hand processor. Add mixed herbs. Serve.

Lentil and Tomato Soup

2 cups of red lentils
4 cups boiling water
A handful of chopped spring onions
1 large onion finely chopped
4-6 tomatoes cut into pieces
1 cube vegetable seasoning
1 teaspoon garlic powder
1 teaspoon onion powder

1 dessertspoon chopped parsley
Pour the water in saucepan and add lentils. Bring to the boil and cook lentils on a low heat for 10-15 mins. Add remaining ingredients. Cook for a further 5 mins. Blend with a hand blender and serve.

Savoury Okra

250g (½ lb) okra
½ cup water
1 onion
1 tomato
1 teaspoon mixed herbs
1 teaspoon parsley
¼ stock cube

Wash and cut the ends off the okra. Chop into small circular ½ inch pieces. Place one cup water in frying pan. Peel and cut unions into small pieces and add to water in frying pan. Cut tomatoes into small pieces; add this to pan as well. Add okra and remaining water. Bring to the boil and simmer for 10-15 mins - until tender. Add herbs, stir well and serve .

For variation add red kidney, butter or pinto beans to mixture. Heat through thoroughly. Serve with whole grain rice, yams or sweet potatoes.

Pan Roasted Vegetables

1 medium sized aubergine
1 medium sized courgette
2 tablespoons wholewheat flour
1 tablespoon vegan bouillon powder
1 teaspoon garlic powder
1 teaspoon onion granule
Juice of ½ a lemon
1 tablespoon parsley
1 cup tomato juice

Wash and cut the vegetables into slim circles. In the meantime place a large frying pan on the stove. Drizzle or better still coat with virgin olive oil. Mix items 3-6 in a small bowl. Coat vegetables on both sides in mixture. Pan roast all vegetables until golden brown. Add tomato juice, parsley and lemon juice. Heat through thoroughly for 2-3 mins. Serve with pasta, rice etc.

Gorgeous Pasta

1 litre of water
250g (½ lb) wholewheat Pasta
1 vegetable stock cube
1 cup tomato juice
1 teaspoon onion powder and 1 teaspoon parsley
1 teaspoon jerk seasoning
1 teaspoon mixed herbs
1 teaspoon garlic powder
1 teaspoon salt (optional)

1 tablespoon sesame seeds (optional)
Juice of ½ lemon (optional)

Place water in medium sized pan and add stock cube. When the water boils, add pasta. Simmer for 20 mins. In the meantime pour tomato juice in a pan; add the remaining ingredients except lemon juice and sesame seeds. Heat thoroughly stirring continually. When pasta is cooked, drain and add to mixture - stir well. Add lemon juice, sesame seeds and stir. Serve.

Variation: Stir in 2 cups thinly sliced cooked green beans and up to 2 cups chickpeas or kidney beans, heat through thoroughly on a low heat, stirring continually.

Baked Sweet Potato

3 medium sweet potatoes

Wash potatoes to remove excess soil. Dry and place in a hot oven gas mark 6 for 40-45 mins until cooked. To test whether cooked or not, insert knife into the centre of the potato. Knife should penetrate easily. Hold potato using an oven glove. Peel and serve with dish of choice. Serves 2 - 3.

Boiled Sweet Potatoes

2 cups (500 mls) 1 pint water
1 teaspoon salt (optional)
250g (½ lb) sweet potatoes - washed and peeled.

Place water in a pan - bring to the boil - add salt and stir. Cut peeled sweet potatoes in 3-4 pieces. Place in a pan.

Bring to boil. Reduce heat and simmer on a low flame for 20 mins or until tender.

Boiled Yam

500g (1 lb) yam
3 cups water
½ teaspoon salt (optional)

Pour water in a saucepan and boil. Peel yam and cut into 3-4 slices. Place yam in boiling water. Bring to boil again. Reduce heat and simmer for 15-20 mins. Serve with tofu dish or similar.

Roast Yam with Orange/Honey Sauce

500g (1 lb) yam - any variety

Place yam on baking tray in hot oven Bake on gas mark 6 for 50-60 mins. Remove and carefully peel. Serve with dish of choice.

To make sauce

1 cup water
1 tablespoon honey
1 onion chopped
2 tomatoes chopped
½ green pepper - cut into strips
Juice of 1 orange and the juice of fi a lemon
1 teaspoon mixed herbs
1 tablespoon soy sauce
2 tablespoons cornflour

Place water in a saucepan and add onion and tomatoes. When tender add the remaining ingredients. Stir well. Bring to the boil and simmer for 2-3 mins. Mix cornflour in a little water and stir into mixture. When thickened, remove from the heat. Cut yam into slices, then cut in halves and place in a serving bowl. Pour sauce over yam. Serve hot, - delicious with a range of hot and cold vegetables.

Boiled Green Bananas

Pour 1 pint of water in a saucepan. Add a little salt - optional. Bring to the boil

In the meantime cut ends off the 2-3 green bananas and slit them vertical back and front. Place the bananas in a deep bowl and cover with boiling water. Leave until skin turns black. Drain off water. Hold bananas with an oven glove or similar and remove peel. Then place bananas in pan of boiling water on the stove and bring to the boil again. Simmer for 20 mins or until tender. Carefully remove bananas from the pan and serve with favourite dish.

Roast Breadfruit

½ -1 whole breadfruit

Place breadfruit in a hot oven gas mark 6 and bake for 50-60 mins or until flesh can be penetrated with a knife. Remove from oven using oven glove or similar. Remove the exposed ends of the breadfruit, as these tend to become crisp during the baking process. Peel and serve with sweet and sour tofu.

Breadfruit Casserole

250g (½ lb) breadfruit
2 carrots
½ vegetable stock cube
2 cups cooked red kidney beans

2 parsnips
1 tomato
3½ cups water
3 sprigs of spring onions
1 teaspoon parsley
1 teaspoon dill top
1 teaspoon rosemary
1 teaspoon onion granules
1 teaspoon garlic powder
Juice of ½ a lemon
1 teaspoon salt (optional)

Peel and slice the breadfruit into thin slices (about 4-5). Remove the core, rather like removing an apple core. Cut each slice into 3-5 pieces. Peel carrots and parsnips and cut into small pieces. Cut tomato finely. Place water in a saucepan. Add parsley, stock cube, rosemary, onion granules and garlic powder. Stir well. Add the remaining ingredients. Bring to the boil, lower heat and simmer for 15 mins. Add spring onions and kidney beans. Bring to the boil again and simmer for a further 7-10 mins or until all vegetables are tender. Mix 1 tablespoon of cornflour in a little water. Add lemon juice mixture. Stir and leave to simmer for 2-3 mins. Stir and serve with a range of vegetables.

Spring Cabbage

1 onion cut finely
A handful of finely chopped spring onion
500g (1 lb) spring cabbage
1 ½ cups boiling water
1 teaspoon onion powder
1 teaspoon garlic powder
1 teaspoon vegan bouillon powder
1 teaspoon each of rosemary, sage, thyme and basil

In a medium sized pan, place half boiling water and add the onions. When soft add the cabbage. Cook on a low heat until tender - stirring occasionally. Add the remaining ingredients, stir and serve.

Cabbage Supreme

1 small head of cabbage
1 cup water
1 onion chopped
2-3 cups cooked black-eyed beans
1 teaspoon salt
1 tablespoon thyme

Shred cabbage as if preparing for coleslaw. Add onion and salt and simmer in water on a low heat. When tender add black-eyed beans. Simmer for 5-8 mins. Add thyme, stir and serve.

Pumpkin Cascade

3-4 good slices of green skinned pumpkin enough for up to 2 people
2 cups water
2 courgettes washed and cut into slices
2 sprigs of spring onions
1 small tin chopped tomato
1 onion chopped
1 red pepper chopped
1 teaspoon mixed herbs
1 teaspoon garlic paste
1 tablespoon tomato puree
1 teaspoon vegan bouillon powder (available from Sainsbury/Tesco).
1-2 tablespoons wholewheat flour
A dash of soy sauce.

Wrap pumpkin in foil and place in a medium oven gas mark 6 for 20-30 mins until tender.

Prepare topping

Place 1 cup water in frying pan. Chop spring onions place in pan. Add chopped onions - simmer on low heat until tender. Add the remaining water, tomatoes chopped pepper, bouillon powder, garlic powder and courgettes - simmer until courgettes are cooked. Add tomato puree - simmer for 5 mins - add a little more water if necessary. Sprinkle in 1-2 tablespoons wholewheat flour, stir and simmer for 2 mins. Add a dash of soy sauce. Scoop pumpkin from skin -

place on a large plate. Pour vegetable mix over pumpkin. Serve.

Cornmeal - Wonder

3 medium sized carrots
1 litre water
2 cups frozen mixed vegetables
1-2 cloves of garlic
1 green pepper
½ cup desiccated coconut
1 parsnip
1½ cups fine cornmeal
1 medium onion cut into segments
2 teaspoons vegan bouillon powder (available from Sainsbury/Tesco)
1 teaspoon mixed herbs and fi teaspoon salt (optional)

In a blender place 100 mls water. Add garlic, pepper and onion pieces, parsnip, carrot and blend until nearly smooth. Pour mixture into saucepan - Add vegetables and coconut and mixed herbs. Add 700 mls water - boil and simmer for 3 mins. Place cornmeal in a bowl - mix slowly with remaining water. Add to mixture in saucepan - bring to the boil stirring continually until mixture thickens. Cover and simmer for 15-20 mins stirring occasionally. Wet interior of small individual serving bowls or large bowl with warm water. Pour mixture into bowls. Leave to stand for 1-2 mins. Turn out onto serving plate and serve with a range of cooked vegetables and side salad.

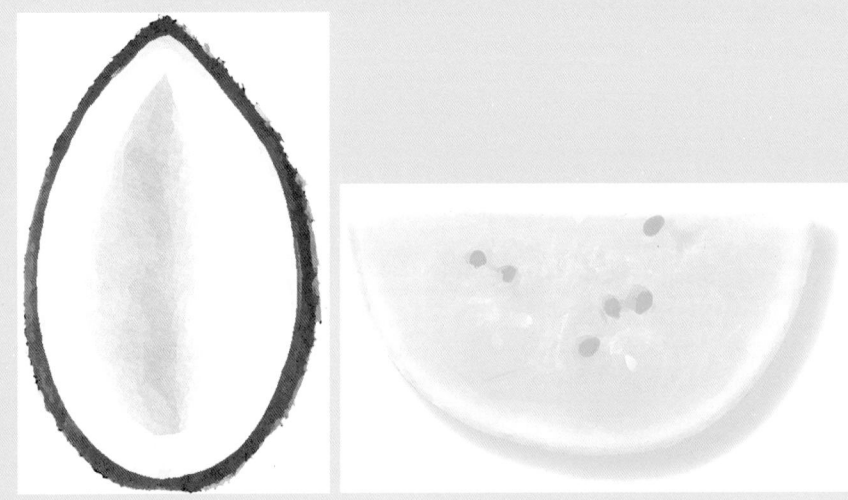

Breakfast Foods

Easy Porridge

1 cup unsweetened soya milk
½ cup oats
½ cup bran flakes
1 well-ripened plum - cut finely
1 dessertspoon raisins and 1-2 dates - chopped finely
Place soya milk and oats in a bowl. Place in microwave for 2 mins. Mix remaining ingredients together and sprinkle on top of porridge.

Millet Surprise

(Millet is available from health food stores)
1 cup millet flakes
2 dates - chopped finely
4 cups soya milk (unsweetened)
1 teaspoon vanilla
Pinch of salt
1 apple chopped

Place millet, dates, salt and milk into pan. Bring to the boil. Simmer on low heat for 20 mins. Stir occasionally and add more milk if necessary. Pour into serving bowl. Top with chopped apples.

Fruity Millet

1 cup millet flakes
1 teaspoon vanilla
4 cups soya milk (unsweetened)

Pinch of salt
1 x 250g tin peaches in own juice - drained and chopped
1-2 tablespoons of 'Eat Natural' a roasted blend of nuts with fruits and honey - available from Tesco.

Place millet, salt and milk into pan, bring to the boil. Simmer on low heat for 15 minutes. Stir occasionally; add more milk if necessary. Add chopped peachess and cook for a further 5 minutes. Pour into serving bowl. Top with 'Eat Natural'.

Nutty Millet Sunrise

1 cup millet flakes
2 dates chopped finely
4 cups soya milk (unsweetened)
1 teaspoon vanilla essence
Pinch of salt
½ cup raisins
¼ cup roughly chopped walnuts
½ chopped fruits e.g. pears apples bananas

Place millet, dates, salt and milk into pan bring to the boil. Simmer on low heat for 20 minutes. Stir occasionally. Add more milk if necessary. Add walnuts and raisins. Pour into serving bowl. When cold turn out onto serving plate Top with favourite soft fruits.

Mango Millet

2 cups soya milk (unsweetened)
1 cup oats

½ cup millet rice - cook as on page 76
½ cup bran flakes
½ peeled chopped mango (top slice only) cut into small pieces.
A few chopped nuts - top with last three ingredients

Coconut Millet

4 cups soya milk
1 cup millet
1 teaspoon vanilla essence
½ peeled chopped mango (top slice only) cut into small pieces
1 teaspoon honey
Pinch salt
1 tablespoon unsweetened desiccated coconut or 1 tablespoon roughly chopped walnuts or sesame seeds

Pour milk in a small saucepan. Add vanilla, salt honey and millet. Stir continually until the mixture begins to boil, simmer on low heat for 20 mins. Serve and top with chopped mango and coconut or sesame seeds.

Barley Combo

(Barley is available from health food stores)
700 mls soya milk
2 pitted dates, chopped finely
1 cup barley
½ teaspoon salt

1 dessertspoon honey
½ cup chopped fruit per person e.g. mangoes, apples, pears.

Place barley in medium saucepan. Add milk and salt. Bring to the boil; simmer for 1-1½ hours, adding more milk as necessary. When barley is soft and tender, add honey or raisin and dates- stir - add more milk if necessary and bring to the boil - stirring all the time. Pour into serving bowls. Top with soft fruits.

Fruity Cornmeal Porridge

1 litre unsweetened soya milk in a saucepan boiled
200 mls additional soya milk
¾ cup finely ground cornmeal
½ cup desiccated coconut
1 teaspoon vanilla essence
1 dessertspoon chopped walnuts
½ teaspoon salt

Mix cornmeal in 200 mls of milk. Add to boiled milk stirring continually. Add vanilla and salt. Return to stove and bring to the boil again - keep stirring. Once thickened add coconut - bring to the boil again. Simmer on a low heat for 10 mins. Mix fruits, nuts and dates together. Pour porridge into bowls and top with mixed fruits and dates. Serves 2-3.

Topping for each person:

1 cup soft fruits (if frozen add 1 tablespoon of water and

simmer on a low heat for 2 mins)
2 dates finely chopped.

Cream of Banana Porridge

2 green bananas
1 cup unsweetened soya milk
2-3 dates chopped finely
pinch of salt
1 teaspoon vanilla essence

Remove both ends from the banana using a vegetable knife. Cut through the skin of each side of the bananas vertically. This makes them easier to peel. Place both bananas in a deep bowl and cover with boiling water until skins blacken. Drain away water and peel. You should be able to remove the skins easily, if not, use a vegetable knife to assist you. Grate bananas using the large serrated edge on the grater. Pour the milk in a saucepan and add the grated bananas. Add the remaining ingredients. Bring mixture to the boil, stirring often. Reduce heat and simmer for 10 mins.

Continue to use:

- Weetabix
- Shredded Wheat
- All-Bran
- Bran Flakes
- Or any other whole grain cereal

topped with fruits in soya or rice milk

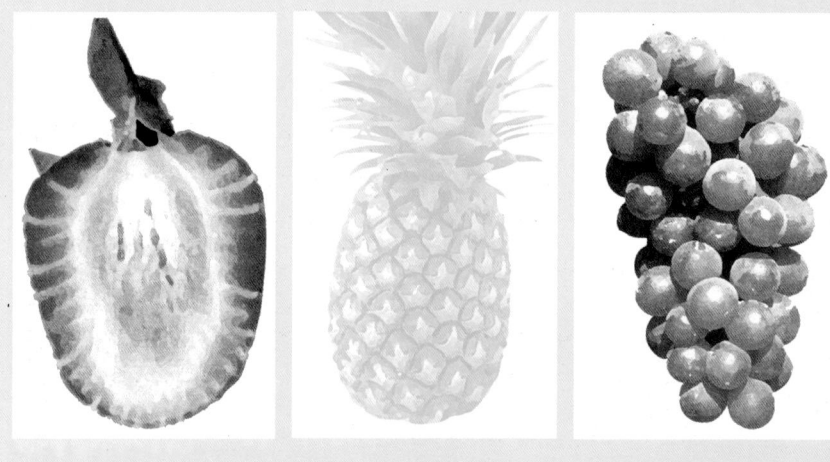

Desserts

Muesli Bake

4 cups muesli
1 cup oats
1 cup chopped walnuts
1 tin peaches in own juice chopped or fruit cocktail in own juice (250g) around 400g with juice
1 teaspoon vanilla
1 cup raisins
1 cup soya milk
Juice of ½ a lemon
1 tablespoon honey

Place all ingredients in a bowl except honey and lemon. Mix well. You may need to add a little more soya milk. The mixture should not be soggy - but should hold together. Pour mixture on a greased baking tray. Bake at gas mark 6 for 45-60 mins, remove from oven. Mix lemon and honey together. Brush the top of cake with mixture. Cover with foil and leave to stand for 10-15 mins. Cut into sections and serve hot - with tofu cream (available from Tesco).

Pumpkin Bakes

2 cups cooked pumpkin
½ cup oatmeal
½ cup Quaker oats
¾ cup raisins
½ cup flaked coconut

1 teaspoon vanilla essence
½ teaspoon salt (optional)

10 dates chopped finely

Place all ingredients in a bowl. Mix well so the ingredients are dispersed evenly. Cover and leave to stand for 10 mins. Place spoonfuls in a 12 sectioned baking tray. Bake at gas mark 6 for 30 mins. Cool and serve - these cakes are firmer if left to cool or served cold.

Walnut Pancakes

1 cup of chopped walnuts
1 cup oats
2 well ripened bananas
3 cups of soya milk
4 pitted dates chopped
1 cup of raisins
$1/2$ - 1 teaspoon lemon juice

Mash bananas in a bowl. Add the remaining ingredients and mix well - add more milk if necessary. Lightly grease a frying pan and place 1 tablespoon full of mixture at a time in pan. Cook for 2-3 mins - turn - press to flatten. Sprinkle with lemon juice. Serve hot or cold.

Cornmeal and Sweet Potato Pudding

1 cup cornmeal
3 cups unsweetened soya milk
10-12 dates - de-stoned and chopped
$1/2$ cup raisins
$1/2$ cup unsweetened desiccated coconut

500g (1 lb) sweet potatoes
Juice of ½ lemon
1 teaspoon orange rind
½ teaspoon salt
1 teaspoon vanilla essence
1 tablespoon honey

Wash peel and grate sweet potato in a mixing bowl. Add raisin, coconut, dates, and orange rind. Mix well. Place 2 cups of soya milk in a pan. Place on a low heat. Mix corn meal in a bowl with remaining milk. Add to milk in pan and bring to boil. Stir occasionally to prevent lumps forming. To this mixture add salt, lemon juice and vanilla essence. When thickened, remove from heat and add to sweet potato mixture in the bowl. Stir well to ensure that the ingredients are evenly dispersed. Stir in honey. Pour mixture in a lightly greased loaf tin. Place in oven gas mark 6 and bake for 1 hr. Leave to stand for about an hour or until very cool. Carefully turn unto a plate. Slice and serve.

Plantain and Sweet Potato Bake

250g (½ lb) cooked sweet mashed potatoes
1 medium size plantain
½ cup unsweetened soya milk
½ cup Quaker oats
½ cup raisins
¼ cup walnuts
1 teaspoon vanilla
Juice of ½ lemon
8-10 dates chopped

Mash sweet potato pieces with a fork. Peel plantain and grater using large grating edge. Add milk and vanilla essence. Mix well together and add cup oats. Mix well. Add chopped walnuts and dates, stir in raisins. Add 1 tablespoon honey. Mix well together. Pour mixture into lightly greased flan case. Bake at gas mark 5 for 30 mins. Brush with lemon juice. Serve hot or cold.

Plantain Oven Bakes

2 cups wholewheat flour
2 cups oatmeal
¼ cup ground walnuts
½ teaspoon salt
1 ripe plantain - grated
6 de-stoned dates, chopped finely
1 eating apple - peeled and cored
½-1 cup warm water
2-3 tablespoons yeast

In a large mixing bowl, place the first 6 ingredients - mix well. Add the grated plantain and chopped dates. Place finely cut eating apple in a pan with a little water - simmer until softened. Add apple to the mixture in the bowl. Add yeast to the cup of boiling water and mix well. Add to mixture in the bowl. Knead well for 3 minutes; divide into 10-12 equal parts. Form into small round shapes. Place on lightly greased baking tray and put somewhere warm to rise overnight. Bake at gas mark 5 for 30 -35 minutes. Serve hot.

Brazil and Apple Bakes

1 cups oats
12 chopped Brazil nuts
2 bananas
6-8 pitted dates
3 cups of soya milk,
1 apple grated
1 cup of raisins
Juice of ½-1 lemon

Place milk in a blender, add dates and blend for a few seconds. Add bananas. Pour mixture into a bowl. Add the remaining ingredients and mix well. Lightly grease a bun tins - makes 4-5 small buns. Place in a hot oven. Cook for 35 mins Gas Mark 6. Sprinkle with lemon juice. Serve hot or cold.

*Basic Pie Crust

2 ¼ cups bran flakes
¾ cup unsweetened desiccated coconut
5-6 tablespoons concentrated fruit juice

Process first two ingredients in a blender. Turn into a mixing bowl. Add fruit juice. Mix evenly. Place in a lightly greased 9-11 inch pie flan case. Press into place evenly with hands. Bake at gas mark 6 for 7-10 mins - until golden brown. For savoury recipe substitute ground almonds for coconut

Filling: 6 golden delicious apples

1-1 ½ cups apple juice
½ cup raisins
6-8 dates, chopped finely
2 tablespoons cornflour
½ tablespoon cold water

Cook first 4 ingredients in a pan until apples are tender. Mix cornflour in water and add to saucepan. Cover on a low heat, stir gently until thickened and liquid is clear. Pour into flan case. Serve hot or cold.
Or: 1 tin sliced peaches in fruit juice, ½ cup raisins and 1 tin fruit salad in fruit juice. 2 tablespoons cornflour. Place fruits, and juices in a pan. Bring to the boil. Stir gently. Mix corn flour in a little water. Add to mixture in pan. Stir well. Cook until mixture thickens and is clear. Pour into flan case. Serve hot or cold with tofu cream, available from Tesco, or cashew cream - see page 87.

Apple and Yam Bake

2 large eating apples
500g (1 lb) yam
Juice of 1-2 lemons
2 cups orange juice
1 cup raisins
1 teaspoon coriander

Place the orange juice in a saucepan. Peel and cut the yam into small pieces. Peal and cut the apple into small pieces. Add to orange juice in the saucepan. Add remaining ingredi ents. Bring to the boil; reduce heat and leave to simmer for 7-10 mins. Remove from the heat and mash together with a fork or potato masher. Scoop into an airtight containing, cool and keep refrigerated.

*Cashew Cream

1 cup water
¾ cup raw cashews
1 tablespoon honey
½ teaspoon vanilla
Pinch of salt

Process first three ingredients until smooth. Pour in a saucepan and bring to the boil. Reduce heat and simmer until thickened. Stir constantly. Add remaining ingredients. Serve hot or cold.

Apricot Wedges

10 dried apricots - cut finely
1 cup Quaker oats
1 cup bran flakes
½ cup chopped walnuts
½ cup pineapple juice - concentrated
Juice of ½ a lemon

Mix all ingredients together in a bowl. Lightly grease a 7-9 inch flan tin. Press mixture in tin. Bake at gas mark 5 for 15-20 mins (should be firm) Sprinkle top with lemon juice.

Leave to cool. Cut into wedges and serve.

Pineapple Scream

1 cup unsweetened soya milk
1 small tin peaches in juice, cut into pieces
1 large tin pineapple
½ cup raisins / dates and walnuts mixed together
1 tablespoon honey
2 cups tofu light (from Sainsbury)
1 sachet vegetable gel (available from Sainsbury or Tesco) mixed in a little warm water

Place all ingredients in a blender except honey, nuts, dates and raisins. Blend until smooth. Pour into saucepan - heat until boiling point is reached. Remove and pour into serving dishes. Top with raisins, nuts and dates. Place in a freezer compartment until set. Remove, drizzle top with honey and serve.

Cornmeal-Supreme

1 cup of cornmeal
1 cup raisins
1 cup shredded unsweetened coconut
1 small tin chopped pineapples
1 teaspoon vanilla
½ cup orange juice
1 teaspoon salt
Tofu cream (available from Tesco)

Mix cornmeal with some of the water until smooth. Add remaining water. Bring to the boil - stir until thickened - add remaining ingredients except orange juice. Stir well - cook for a further 2 mins on a low heat stirring continually. Pour mixture into greased cake / loaf tin. Pour orange juice on top. Bake at gas mark 6 for 45-60 mins. Leave to stand until cool / cold. Turn out unto a plate. Slice and serve with tofu cream.

Fruity Ice cream

2 cups frozen Black Forest fruits (from Tesco)
3 frozen bananas
½ - 1 cup concentrated pineapple juice

Place all fruits in a blender. Add pineapple juice slowly and blend until smooth. Turn mixture out into a bowl. Serve as ice cream substitute.

Raspberry Ice cream

2 cups frozen raspberries
3 frozen bananas
½ - 1 cup concentrated orange juice

Place all fruits in a blender. Add orange juice slowly and blend until smooth. Turn mixture out into a bowl. Serve as ice cream substitute.

Strawberry Ice cream

2 cups frozen strawberries
2-3 frozen bananas
½ - 1 cup concentrated orange juice

Place all fruits in a blender. Add orange juice slowly and blend until smooth. Turn mixture out into a bowl. Serve as ice cream substitute.

Banana Smoothie

2-3 bananas
1 cup strawberries
1 - 1 ½ cups milk
1 teaspoon vanilla essence

Blend ingredients together in a blender. Pour into small glasses. Top with chopped strawberries and serve.

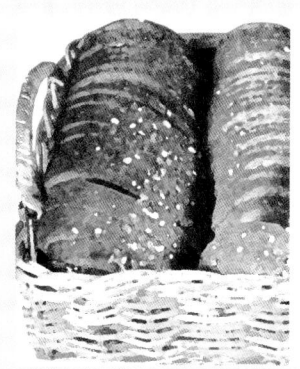

Walnut Date Spread

1 cup water
15 dates chopped finely
1 cup walnuts
Use the same dry cup for all ingredients.

Blend ingredients for 1 minute, until smooth. Makes a delicious butter/margarine substitute.

*Orange Cashew Spread

1 cup cashews
1 cup raisins
1 cup concentrated orange juice

Place all ingredients in a blender and blend until smooth. Use instead of jam or marmalade.

* Raisin-Coconut Sandwich Filling or Spread

2 cups raisins
1 cup coconut
1 teaspoon vanilla essence

Blend on low speed half of each ingredient at a time. Add a little of your favourite cereal milk for blending.

*Walnut-Herb Butter

1 cup water, 1 cup walnuts
1-2 cloves garlic

1 tablespoon onion powder
1 tablespoon lemon juice
1 tablespoon parsley
¼ teaspoon thyme
½ teaspoon salt

Liquify in the blender all the ingredients but the herbs, crumbling them in last. Add salt gradually, to taste. You may use as a spread on bread.

* Cashew Cheese

1 chopped red capsicum
3 tablespoons brewer's yeast
¾ cup cashews
1 teaspoon garlic powder
2 tablespoons sesame seeds
½ - 1 cup water
½ teaspoon salt
¾ cup lemon juice

Blend all ingredients on low speed, adding the water gradually and increasing to high speed until very smooth. Delicious as a spread on bread, potatoes, sandwiches, Substitute for cheese in any recipe except where grated or sliced cheese is needed.

Sandwich Spread

2-3 sprigs spring onion
1 tablespoon chopped parsley

1 x 250g tin of red beans
1 teaspoon bouillon powder

Crush beans with a fork; add parsley, onion bouillon powder - available from Tesco. Store in fridge in airtight container. Use as spread on bread, wholemeal crackers, oatcakes etc.

*Date-Nut Spread

2 cups cut up pitted dates
1-1½ cups water

Simmer these gently for 15-20 mins, then remove from stove and stir to a paste. Mash any chunks. Add 1 cup chopped walnuts or pecans. Variation: Blend date pieces and walnuts in blender with a little water on low speed.
For orange Date-Nut Spread: Add finely grated orange rind to the above ingredients.

* Tomato Ketchup

1 8oz can tomato sauce
½ cup sunflower seeds
½ teaspoon basil
Pinch of oregano
Juice of ½ lemon (to taste)
Sprinkle salt

Pour can of sauce into blender jar. Add seeds and all other ingredients except lemon juice. Blend on low speed till very smooth. May add a few drops of water or lemon juice according to the taste of the cook!

* Tofu Sour Cream or Mayonnaise

1 (250g) block regular tofu,
2 teaspoons onion powder
½ cup fresh lemon juice
½ teaspoon dill weed
1 clove garlic
½ teaspoon salt

Blend all ingredients until very smooth. Add a little water for blending if necessary. For a more 'blue cheese' type of taste, add the greater amount of dill. Keep refrigerated in an airtight container.

*Tofu Mayonnaise

1 (250 g) block tofu, drained and rinsed
1 teaspoon onion powder
¼ cup water
¾ cup lemon juice
½ teaspoon salt
1 cup raw cashews
2 tablespoons honey

Liquify tofu with water until blended. Add remaining ingredients and blend until creamy.

* Tofu Sour Cream

1 block (250g) tofu
½ cup fresh lemon juice

1 clove garlic
2 teaspoons onion powder
½ teaspoon dill weed
½ teaspoon salt

Blend all ingredients until very smooth. Add a little water for blending if necessary. Keep refrigerated in an airtight container. Yields two cups or 32 servings

Houmous

1½ cups cooked chickpeas
1 teaspoon onion granules
1 teaspoon garlic powder
Juice of 1 lemon
1 tablespoon water or unsweetened soya milk
1 tablespoon sesame seeds (optional)
Pinch of salt

Place all ingredients in a blender and liquefy until mixture is completely smooth. (A small nut chopper seems to work well). Place in an airtight container and keep refrigerated. Makes a delicious filling for wholemeal pitta bread with a range of salad vegetables.

Guacamole

1 avocado pear - peel and de-stoned
1 tomato chopped
Juice of ½ a lemon
½ teaspoon onion powder
½ teaspoon garlic powder

Mash avocado pear in a bowl. Cut tomatoes into very tiny pieces. Add lemon juice and remaining ingredients. Mix well and serve. Delicious as sandwich filling with salad.

Salsa Dip/Pasta Sauce

1 ½ cups tomato juice
2 teaspoons parsley
2 teaspoons oregano
2 tablespoons lemon juice
½-1 teaspoon vegan buollion powder
2 teaspoons garlic powder
1 heaped tablespoon wholewheat flour

Pour tomato sauce in a small saucepan. Slowly add the flour, stirring continually. Add the remaining ingredients. Use as a dip or pour over wholewheat pasta.

Corn, Cashew and Walnut Pate

½ cup walnuts
½ cup cashews
1 red pepper - cut thinly
1 x 250g tin sweet corn
A squeeze of lemon juice, salt to taste

Place nuts in a blender and grind finely. Add chopped pepper and blend until pepper is well dispersed. Drain corn well and add to mixture in blender. Blend until mixture is nearly smooth. Pour into a bowl and add salt and /or lemon juice to taste. Serve on wholemeal bread or oatmeal crackers.

References

Barnard N. et al. (2003) Acceptability of a Low Fat Vegan Diet Compares Favourably to a Step 1 Diet in a Randomised Controlled Trial. Diabetes 52 (1) 556.

Crane M G Sample C **Regression of Diabetic Neuropathy with Total Vegetarian Diet in Journal of Nutritional Medicine** 1994, 4, 431-43

Diabetes UK - www.diabetes.org.uk/diabetes/under.htm

Department of Health (DOH) (2002) **National Service Framework for Diabetes.** Department of Health, London, England.

Food and Agriculture Organisation/World Health Organisation (FAO/WHO) Joint Report (2003). **Diet, Nutrition and the Prevention of Chronic Diseases,** WHO Geneva, www.FAO.org.

Internal Diabetic Foundation (IDF) (2003) **Diabetes Facts and Figures.** Available from: www.idf.org/home/index.cfm?node=6

Teske M M D **How It Works -Diabetes Is Reversible!** By www.reversingdiabetes.org/?page=hiw

National Journal of Medicine (2003) **Position of the American Dietetic** Association and Dieticians of Canada: Vegetarian Diets. Journal of American Diet Association. 103, 748-765.

Nedley N (1999) **Proof Positive Quality Books** Inc USA

Nicholson A.S. et al. (1999) Towards improved Management of NIDDM: **A Randomised Controlled Pilot Intervention Using a Low Fat, Vegetarian Diet.** Preventative Medicine. 29, 87-91.

Pusey V. (1995) Advising Afro Caribbeans on diet and diabetes Nurse Prescriber/Community Nurse Dec 1995 – 28-30

The HB A1C
www.//medweb.bham.ac.uk/easdec/prevention/what_is_the_hba1c.htm #hba

The Weimar institute, California USA -
www.reversingdiabetes.org OR **www.weimar.org**

World Health Organization (WHO) (2002) The Cost of Diabetes Fact Sheet No. 236. Available from:
www.who.int/mediacentre/factsheets/fs236/en

World Health Organization (WHO) (2003) **Diet Nutrition and Prevention of Chronic Diseases.** WHO, Geneva

Notes

Notes

Notes

Notes

Notes

Notes

Notes